Najla BAHLOUL

Treatment of cancer pain in the elderly

Najla BAHLOUL

Treatment of cancer pain in the elderly

ScienciaScripts

Imprint

Cover image: www.ingimage.com

This book is a translation from the original published under ISBN 978-620-6-72435-3.

Publisher:
Sciencia Scripts
is a trademark of
Dodo Books Indian Ocean Ltd. and OmniScriptum S.R.L publishing group

120 High Road, East Finchley, London, N2 9ED, United Kingdom
Str. Armeneasca 28/1, office 1, Chisinau MD-2012, Republic of Moldova, Europe
Printed at: see last page
ISBN: 978-620-8-31110-0

TREATMENT OF THE CANCER PAIN IN THE ELDERLY

1.INTRODUCTION

Despite its many adverse consequences on the functioning, emotional health and quality of life of those who suffer from it, pain remains under-treated in the elderly, in all care settings [1]. Only 34% of older people living at home with ongoing pain receive an analgesic, of whom only 9% are treated with an opioid [1]. Elderly patients with musculoskeletal pain are more likely to be treated with a non-steroidal anti-inflammatory drug (NSAID) and less likely to receive an opioid than younger patients with similar pain [2].Elderly patients are also less likely to receive analgesics when presenting to the emergency department [3] or as outpatients [2] or post-operatively for hip fractures [4]. The problem is even more acute in nursing homes for the elderly, where around 25% of patients with ongoing pain receive no analgesic at all [5, 6], 16% are treated with a "weak" opioid and only 3% receive a "strong" opioid [6]. When they are prescribed, analgesics are often given "as required" despite the presence of ongoing pain [6].very elderly patients and those with cognitive deficits are at greater risk of sub-optimal treatment of their pain [1,4, 5].with ageing, pain may contribute to a progressive decline in physiological reserve and increased frailty [7].

Persistent pain may be associated with impaired physical function, falls, anorexia, sleep disturbance, depression and anxiety, agitation and delirium, and impaired cognitive function [8].

On the other hand, many elderly people function well despite persistent pain, and the degree to which pain interacts with their function is largely related to biopsychosocial comorbidities [9].

2.GENERAL APPROACH

Persistent pain is defined as pain that persists beyond the expected healing time, or for at least three to six months [10]. Older people may under-report the severity of pain due to misconceptions that pain is an integral part of ageing [11] or fears of dependency [12]. The coexistence of sensory (e.g. visual and/or hearing impairment) and/or cognitive impairments can also complicate pain assessment in the elderly patient.

2.1.Questioning

Prescribing an effective treatment begins with an interview which :
- defines the parameters affected by pain and the severity of their impact;

- highlights the main comorbidities that contribute to pain or influence the effects of treatment;

- identifies the treatment objectives [13].

The interview identifies the main medical, psychological and social co-morbidities that may contribute to the pain and/or have an impact on the response to treatment.

It is essential to document accurately and comprehensively the impact of pain on the function of the older person. Answers to the following questions will help determine the impact of pain in the older person and, therefore, the key outcomes of treatment [14] :

- How bad is your pain (now, worse or average) compared with last week?

- How many days in the past week have you been unable to do any of the following?

What would you like to do about your pain?

- Over the past week, how often has pain interfered with your ability to take care of yourself, for example, bathing, eating, dressing and using the toilet?

- Over the past week, how often has pain affected your ability to carry out household tasks such as shopping, preparing meals, paying bills and driving?

- How often do you take part in enjoyable activities such as getting together with friends or travelling?

- Over the past week, how often did pain interfere with these activities?

- Over the past week, how often has your pain interfered with your ability to exercise?

- Does pain interfere with your ability to think clearly?

- Does the pain interfere with your appetite? Have you lost weight?

- Does the pain interfere with your sleep? How many times in the past week?

- Has the pain affected your energy, your mood, your personality or your relationships with others?

- In the past week, how often have you taken painkillers?

- How would you rate your health at the moment? Excellent, good, fair or poor?

2.2. Physical examination

As well as assessing standard vital signs (temperature, blood pressure, respiratory rate, pulse), cognitive function and mobility and balance should be assessed in elderly patients with persistent pain. Assessment of mobility is important because of the possibility of falls caused by pain or certain analgesics.

2.3.Imaging

Degenerative pathology is common in elderly patients with or without pain [15]. Consequently, radiological examinations should be limited to patients in whom the questioning and physical examination suggest a disease requiring specialist intervention (osteoarthritis of the hip, narrow lumbar canal).

2.4.Identification of physical factors contributing to persistent pain

A fundamental principle of geriatric medicine is that the pathology may make the patient vulnerable to other stressors and that these stressors may be the targets of treatment rather than the pathology itself [16]. For example, a patient with low back pain may have a degenerative spinal disease, but the target of treatment may be coexisting depression.

Myofascial pain, chronic low back pain, narrow lumbar canal and fibromyalgia are the most common and misdiagnosed conditions that cause persistent pain in the elderly. Persistent pain in the elderly is often generalised. Generalized osteoarthritis and fibromyalgia are two common causes of generalized pain in this age group. age. History and physical examination may help in differential diagnosis with other multifocal pain disorders common in the elderly [17]. No randomised trials examining the efficacy of fibromyalgia treatment have been conducted exclusively in the elderly.

3.SPECIFIC ASPECTS OF PAIN MANAGEMENT IN THE ELDERLY

In order to treat pain in the elderly appropriately, it is important to be familiar with the pharmacological changes associated with ageing, as well as the specific changes in the pharmacology of different analgesics. Ageing is associated with a number of pharmacokinetic and pharmacodynamic changes. These changes usually begin gradually, but should always be considered when prescribing drugs to patients over the age of 70.

3.1. Pharmacokinetic changes

Data on age-related pharmacokinetic changes are limited, but some changes have been consistently reported by several authors. Although most studies have been carried out in healthy elderly subjects, some studies suggest that pharmacokinetic and pharmacodynamic changes are more significant in frail elderly subjects than in healthy elderly subjects [18].

3.1.1. Absorption

***a*-Oral absorption**

Gastric secretion decreases with ageing in approximately 25% of subjects aged over 50, leading to an increase in gastric pH. Decreases in gastrointestinal motility, splanchnic blood flow, the number of active transporters and absorption surface area have also been reported [19]. Other factors, often encountered in elderly patients, may influence the oral absorption of drugs: comorbidities, drugs that slow gastrointestinal transit, constipation, chronic use of laxatives, gastro-oesophageal reflux and dysphagia [18, 20]. A slowing of gastric emptying and an increase in transit time may lead to a delay in reaching maximum plasma concentration for drugs administered in solid form (capsules, tablets), but the fraction absorbed remains the same [21]. Absorption of drugs administered in liquid form is not affected.

b-Rectal absorption

There is currently no evidence to suggest a change in absorption. in the elderly.

c-Transdermal absorption

Ageing is associated with a reduction in the hydration of the stratum corneum, the thickness and elasticity of the skin and subcutaneous tissue. This may increase the function of the stratum corneum as a barrier for water-soluble molecules, but does not affect fat-soluble molecules (e.g. buprenorphine, fentanyl). The bioavailability of drugs administered transdermally is often unpredictable in elderly patients, with significant inter-individual variability [19].

3.1.2. Distribution

Age-related changes in distribution have a major impact on drug pharmacokinetics [19, 22]. The volume of distribution of water-soluble drugs is reduced, which increases their plasma concentration and requires a lower dose. Conversely, the volume of distribution of fat-soluble drugs is increased, which reduces their plasma concentration and prolongs their half-life, often resulting in accumulation [19].

Ageing is also often associated with a reduction in the level of of serum albumin [23], which is more frequent in the presence of chronic disease or malnutrition, and increases the free fraction of the drug. However, these changes are only significant for drugs with a protein binding rate of over 90%, a low volume of distribution and a narrow therapeutic index [24].

3.1.3. Metabolism

Liver mass and blood flow decrease with age, which reduces the clearance of high clearance drugs. Data on low clearance drugs are contradictory, with some studies suggesting a 20-60% decrease in intrinsic metabolic clearance [25]. The activity of phase I enzymatic reactions (oxidation, reduction, hydrolysis) appears to be reduced, while that of phase II reactions (glucuronidation, acetylation, sulphation) is preserved [22, 26]. There is very little data on age-related changes in cytochrome activity, but it does not appear to be significantly altered [20].

3.1.4. Renal excretion

Renal mass and tubular secretion decrease significantly with age. Glomerular filtration decreases by 30-50% at the age of 80, leading to an accumulation of drugs excreted by the kidneys. Serum creatinine levels are not a reliable indicator of renal function in the elderly due to a decrease in muscle mass concomitant with a decrease in glomerular filtration [27]. The best way to estimate renal function and creatinine clearance is the Cockroft-Gault formula (albeit imperfect), which takes into account age, weight, serum creatinine and sex [28]. However, in elderly patients who are malnourished and have reduced muscle mass, this formula may also overestimate creatinine clearance.

3.2. Pharmacodynamic changes

The pharmacodynamic changes associated with ageing often result in an increase in the sensitivity of elderly patients to drugs and, consequently, in an increased frequency of adverse effects [29]. More specifically, increased sensitivity of cholinergic receptors makes elderly patients more susceptible to the adverse effects of anticholinergic drugs, including tricyclic antidepressants. A decrease in homeostasis may explain the slower recovery of altered physiological function in elderly patients, including normalisation of renal function or haemoglobin following acute renal failure or gastrointestinal bleeding caused by non-steroidal anti-inflammatory drugs.

4.TREATMENT OBJECTIVES

The primary aim of treating persistent pain is to improve function and quality of life while minimising the adverse effects of treatment. Identifying the impact of pain on all aspects of the patient's life allows the clinician to determine treatment goals and assess the response to treatment in a way that is meaningful to the individual [30]. Because of the multi-dimensional nature of persistent pain, pain disappearance is not a realistic goal. It is therefore important to ensure that the elderly patient understands three general principles in their expectations of optimal pain management:

- Persistent pain is multifactorial, requiring an approach that takes several aetiologies into account and includes pharmacological and non-pharmacological strategies.

- Persistent pain is treatable, with an expected improvement, but it is not curable.

- Although the pain is not completely relieved, a substantial improvement in function is realistic [17].

Effective pain management must take into account not only the underlying condition(s) contributing to the pain, but also the patient's comorbidities, the increased potential for drug interactions, and environmental factors: physical, psychosocial and economic.

5.NON-PHARMACOLOGICAL TREATMENTS

Non-drug techniques are recommended in synergy with drug therapy in elderly patients. This multimodal management often avoids risky dosage escalation in this vulnerable population. There have been few studies specifically on the elderly, such as transcutaneous neurostimulation and psychotherapy (in particular cognitive behavioural therapies) [31, 32].

There is also a presumption that acupuncture is effective for pain. postherpetic [33]. The efficacy of hypnosis has been demonstrated in elderly subjects [34] but with a Mini Mental State (MMS) > 25 [35]. A 2018 meta-analysis evaluating psychological interventions (i.e. cognitive behavioural therapy alone or in combination with other therapies) in elderly patients (mean age 72) with chronic pain reported a small reduction in pain sustained over six months [36]. The benefits were greater with group therapy than with individual therapy. The efficacy of non-pharmacological treatments does not appear to differ in older adults compared to other ages. The 2017 American College of Physicians (ACP) recommendations for the treatment of acute, subacute and chronic low back pain (LBP) recommend non-pharmacological treatments early in the treatment of patients with chronic LBP [37, 38].

6.PHARMACOLOGICAL TREATMENT

Pain treatments for the elderly are the same as those for younger patients, but are not always adequately adapted, usually because of a lack of knowledge of age-related pharmacological changes, the pathophysiological mechanisms involved, adverse effects, potential drug interactions, or because pain is not detected and psychotropic drugs are used too quickly, or because the patient does not understand [39].

Analgesics used in the management of pain are classically classified as non-opioids and opioids, in tiers 1, 2 and 3 by the World Health Organisation, and other classifications based on mechanism of action have also been proposed [40]. Co-antalgesics such as antidepressants and antiepileptics are particularly used in the management of neuropathic pain. Non-opioid drugs include paracetamol, non-steroidal anti-inflammatory drugs (NSAIDs), including aspirin and nefopam. Weak" opioids include codeine and tramadol. Level 3 analgesics (strong opioids) are indicated immediately for very intense pain and for moderate to severe pain that does not respond to level 2 analgesics (weak opioids).

6.1. Non-opioid analgesics

6.1.1. Paracetamol

Because of its good efficacy/tolerance ratio, paracetamol is often prescribed as a first-line treatment for mild to moderate pain at a maximum dose of 3 g/day (500 to 1000 mg every 4 to 6 hours) in the elderly, where the prevalence of joint pathologies, particularly osteoarthritis, is very high. In the very elderly or frail, a weight adjustment is necessary: below 50 kg, the maximum dose is 3 g/day and for a weight of 33 kg, the maximum dose is 2 g/day [41]. Recent meta-analyses have cast doubt on its efficacy in chronic pain (osteoarthritis)[42], as well as its tolerability [43, 44].The adverse effects traditionally reported are rare (Table I) [45]. Acute overdose can lead to hepatotoxicity and even irreversible hepatic necrosis, and the antidote for paracetamol is N-acetyl-cysteine. Paracetamol should therefore be administered with caution in cases of malnutrition, prolonged infancy, alcoholism, post-surgery, dehydration, and in cases of known liver disease. However, it remains the analgesic of choice over NSAIDs in the elderly [46]. A fairly recently described adverse effect of paracetamol concerns its interaction with warfarin, with the risk of haemorrhage [47].

The possibility of using the intravenous (IV) route (infusion over 15 minutes) when it is impossible to use the oral route or when the patient has to fast is a good alternative to the 1000 mg dose (3 g per day) [48]. Although the serum peak is faster with IV than with oral administration, the efficacy is the same and it is advisable to switch back to oral administration as soon as possible.

6.1.2. Non-steroidal anti-inflammatory drugs

As a general rule, non-steroidal anti-inflammatory drugs (NSAIDs) should only be used briefly (e.g. one to two weeks) during episodes of increased nociceptive pain [49].When NSAIDs are required in the elderly, the drug should be selected on the basis of risk factors for cardiovascular and gastrointestinal disease. NSAIDs inhibit both isoforms 1 (COX-1) and 2 (COX-2) of cyclooxygenase. Their safety profile therefore depends on the affinity ratio for these two isoforms. Preferential action on COX-1 increases the risk of complications in the digestive tract, and preferential action on COX-2 increases the risk of cardiovascular complications [51]. Thus, the specific effects of NSAIDs in the elderly are on the digestive, cardiac and renal systems, and the risk of confusion needs to be monitored [31]. Dosage should be kept as low as possible for the shortest possible period of time (< 8 days), with creatinine levels checked at D5. Co-administration of NSAIDs with low-dose aspirin, oral anticoagulants and selective serotonin reuptake inhibitors (SSRIs) increases the frequency and severity of gastrointestinal disorders (haemorrhage, ulceration, perforation) [48].

In a 2014 meta-analysis of 280 trials comparing NSAIDs versus placebo and 474 trials comparing NSAIDs, the risk of coronary and vascular events was increased with COX-2 inhibitors, high-dose diclofenac and possibly ibuprofen, but naproxen did not increase this risk [52].

Topical NSAIDs are recommended for osteoarthritis of the knee and hand because they are non-inferior to oral NSAIDs and have a better safety profile. They should not be co-prescribed with oral NSAIDs (Fig. 1) [53]. It should be noted that aspirin for pain relief (WHO recommendation) should not be used in the elderly.

The guidelines of the American Geriatrics Society recommend that NSAIDs should be considered only rarely, and with great caution, in very well selected elderly patients who have not been relieved with other non-opioids. [54]. Proton pump inhibitors should be prescribed in combination with NSAIDs and coxibs when these are used for a long period [54] and elderly patients treated with NSAIDs should be reassessed regularly to ensure efficacy and the absence of toxicity and drug interactions (Table I) [54].

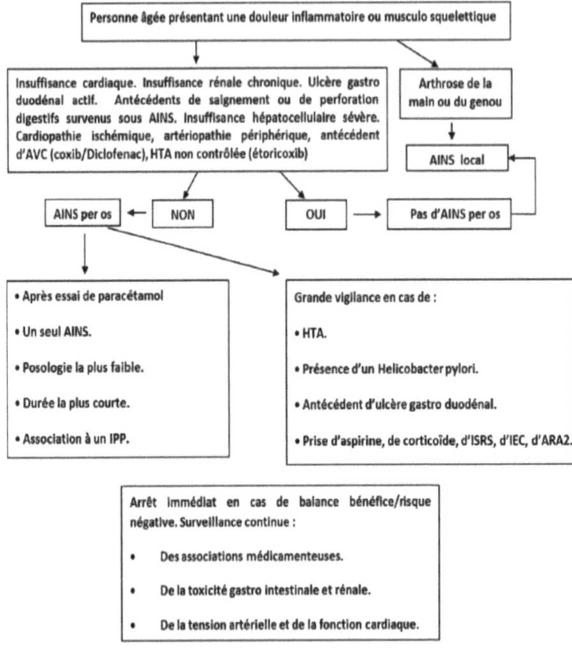

Figure 1: Algorithm for the use of NSAIDs[39].

6.1.3. Nefopam

Nefopam is a non-opioid central analgesic, mainly used in acute situations. It is not recommended for elderly patients [55]. In practice, nefopam is mainly used orally (off-label), on sugar, and there are no studies on this route of administration.

Table I: Most frequent adverse reactions to non-opioid analgesics [45].

Analgésique	Effets indésirables les plus fréquents	Précautions et contre-indications
Non-opioïdes		
Paracétamol	• aucun à dose thérapeutique • risque d'hépatotoxicité si dose maximale quotidienne dépassée • risque d'insuffisance rénale chronique avec utilisation prolongée de hautes doses	• ne pas dépasser 3 000 mg/jour lors d'utilisation prolongée • possibilité d'augmenter jusqu'à 4 000 mg/jour à court terme ou si meilleure réponse qu'avec dose plus faible et enzymes hépatiques vérifiés régulièrement
Anti-inflammatoires non-stéroïdiens (AINS)	• gastriques: ulcère gastrique, gastrite • rénaux : insuffisance rénale aiguë, hyperkaliémie • cardiovasculaires: rétention hydrosodée, insuffisance cardiaque, hypertension artérielle, possible augmentation de la mortalité cardiaque	• si utilisation prolongée, favoriser AINS sélectif pour la COX-2 (célécoxib) • prescrire protection gastrique (inhibiteur de la pompe à protons ou misoprostol) • vérifier la fonction rénale et les électrolytes régulièrement si utilisation prolongée

6.2. Weak opioids

6.2.1. General

After paracetamol, weak opioids are the most commonly prescribed analgesics for the elderly [56, 57]. They are recommended for moderate to severe pain and when paracetamol has failed, particularly in the treatment of chronic non-cancer pain [58]. Their efficacy is comparable and recognised in In geriatric medicine, however, the problem of tolerance frequently leads to discussion of their value compared with low doses of strong opioids. Certain specific rules for prescribing a weak opioid in geriatric medicine should be observed. apply [39]: -The recommended interval between doses for people over 75 should be combined with a reduction in dosage on initiation, using galenic forms with a short half-life;

-All three weak opioids are equally effective in treating nociceptive pain. There is no need to favour one over the other, apart from the usual benefit/risk balance, contraindications and co-prescriptions.

• frequent self-medication with paracetamol should be reported when the product is used weak fixed paracetamol-opioid combinations

• the side-effects are broadly identical to those of strong opioids and are largely dose-dependent; they should therefore be anticipated and prevented, such as constipation and acute urine retention, which are well known in geriatric medicine.

6.2.2. Tramadol

Unlike other opioids, Tramadol has been well studied in elderly subjects. The pharmacokinetic properties of immediate-release and sustained-release formulations do not appear to be significantly altered [59] but, according to one study, patients aged over 75 years require 20% less dose than younger patients for equivalent relief [59]. Both formulations are equally effective and well tolerated in elderly and younger patients [59]. In patients with pain secondary to osteoarthritis of the knee or hip, extended-release tramadol has been reported to be as effective as extended-release diclofenac, with a lower incidence of serious adverse events [60].Secondary effects are mainly the nausea/vomiting dizziness, drowsiness, constipation and orthostatic hypotension [45]. The precautions and contraindications are as follows:

- do not exceed the maximum daily dose of paracetamol if using a tramadol-paracetamol combination

-lowered seizure threshold, so contraindicated in patients with a history of seizures epilepsy

- theoretical risk of serotonin syndrome when used in high doses in combination with other drugs that increase serum serotonin levels (e.g. SSRIs, SNRIs)

-need for withdrawal if switch to opioid

6.2.3. Codeine

Codeine is a pro-drug which requires conversion into its active metabolites (morphine and norcodeine) by cytochrome CYP2D6 in order to exert its analgesic activity. In practice, the large number of formulations combining codeine and paracetamol in varying dosages means that particular care needs to be taken when prescribing them, specifying the desired dose of codeine. A dose of 20mg of codeine is the minimum possible dose to start with in the elderly, taken every 4 to 6 hours, combined with an additional dose of 500mg of paracetamol if efficacy is insufficient and depending on co-morbidities (without exceeding 3g/day of paracetamol). If efficacy is insufficient but tolerance is good, the dosage can be increased to 30 mg of codeine per day. The maximum dose is 180 mg per day, i.e. 60 mg of codeine per dose. The LP form of dihydro-codeine, twice as potent as codeine, is an interesting alternative to repeated doses of codeine after titration [39].

6.3. Strong opioids

As in younger patients, opioids are recommended in elderly patients for the treatment of moderate to severe chronic pain with functional impact or reduced quality of life [54, 61]. When the recommendations for use in the elderly are applied, their good handling and tolerance mean that they are sometimes preferred to weak opioids or NSAIDs [62, 63]. The risk of addiction is lower than in younger patients, and in all cases very low [64, 65].

6.3.1. Available molecules

a- Morphine

Morphine does not show age-related changes in pharmacokinetics [66]. As the active metabolites are eliminated by the kidneys, morphine should be avoided in patients with impaired renal function (GFR <30 mL/min) [66].

It is also necessary to adapt the dosage by titrating the dose using small doses of sustained-release morphine for the background dose and normal-release morphine for acute attacks [39].

b- Oxycodone

Oxycodone is the strong opioid of choice in the elderly because of its short half-life, absence of toxic metabolites and bioavailability, for both short- and long-acting forms [67].

*c-*Transdermal fentanyl

There are greater fluctuations in transcutaneous passage in the elderly, making it more difficult to predict bioavailability [68]. Because of its high liposolubility, fentanyl is eliminated more slowly in the elderly.The transdermal patch may be a good alternative for patients who have difficulty swallowing. Finally, its elimination, which is not linked to the kidney, makes it a molecule of choice in renal failure [63].

d- Hydromorphone

Its pharmacokinetic properties are comparable to those of morphine, but it is better tolerated in cases of renal failure because its metabolites have less affinity for opiate receptors.

*e-*Agonist-antagonist and partial agonist

Buprenorphine is a high-affinity partial mu-opioid receptor agonist that can be used safely in patients with renal failure [69] and is mainly used as a replacement therapy. Nalbuphine is never indicated for chronic pain.

f- Methadone

Because of its lipid solubility and high protein binding, methadone has a large volume of distribution and a long and variable half-life, ranging from 8.5 to 120 hours [70]. These characteristics make dose adjustment methadone, especially in elderly patients with limited reserves, altered hepatic metabolism and impaired renal function. For these reasons, methadone should be started and increased cautiously, by clinicians who are familiar with its use and risks [54].

6.3.2. Choice of opioid and dosage

The choice and dose of opioid depend on the desired route of administration (e.g. oral or transdermal), time to onset of action, duration of action, drug interactions, co-morbidities and susceptibility to side effects (Table II).

The recommended doses for initiating strong opioids [48] :

-15 to 30 mg of oral morphine/day, i.e. between 2.5 and 5 mg per dose every 4 hours (or 6 hours if clearance < 30 ml/min), i.e. 7.5 to 15 mg/day subcutaneously or 5 to 10 mg/day IV; ORAMORPH drop form 1 drop = 1.25 mg,

-10 to 20 mg oxycodone (a slightly higher dose than that given by oxycodone sulphate) morphine) orally/day, 7 to 14 mg/day subcutaneously or IV.

Table II: Summary table of doses and duration of action of compounds [48].

Molécules	Dose initiale per os (PO)	Dose sous-cutanée (SC)/jour	Dose intra-veineuse (IV)/jour	Durée d'action	Délai d'action après dose unique ou 1re administration	Durée du chevauchement avec molécule précédente lors d'un relais
Morphine LI	15 à 30 mg/j	7,5 à 15 mg	5 à 10 mg	4 h	45 min PO et SC	–
Morphine LP	20 mg/j	–	–	12 h	4 h	4 h
Oxycodone LI	10 à 20 mg/j	7 à 14 mg/j	7 à 14 mg/j	4 à 6 h	45 min PO et SC	–
Oxycodone LP	10 à 20 mg/j	–	–	12 h	4 h	4 h
Fentanyl patch	Jamais pour initier palier 3	–	–	72 h	12 h	12 h

In general, reasonable choices for the elderly include morphine, oxycodone, hydromorphone, fentanyl and buprenorphine. The majority of patients suffering from chronic pain will use oral medication. Patients who have difficulty swallowing may benefit from medicines available in liquid form (e.g. hydromorphone, morphine, oxycodone). A transdermal patch (e.g. fentanyl, buprenorphine) may also be a good alternative for patients with difficulty swallowing [68]. As with all long-acting opioids, the patch should be avoided in opioid-naive patients [71]. Patients suffering from continuous pain will benefit from background treatment and the possibility of "rescue" doses in the event of paroxysmal attacks of pain (1/6ème to 1/10ème of the daily dose). This is useful for people with cognitive dysfunction, impaired memory or an unreliable caregiver. Patients taking long-acting opioids may experience episodes of breakthrough pain, for which immediate-acting and long-acting opioids can be used. (e.g. morphine, oxycodone) should be available. Patients with renal impairment should reduce the dose of opioids (hydromorphone, morphine, oxycodone) or take drugs that are not eliminated by the kidneys (buprenorphine, fentanyl, for example). Opioid doses should be reduced in older adults and slowly adjusted accordingly, with close monitoring for side effects. It has been suggested that the initial dose should be reduced by 25% for a 60-year-old patient (50% for an 80-year-old patient) compared with the initial dose normally received by a 40-year-old patient, but at the same intervals [72]. Older adults generally have increased pharmacodynamic sensitivity to opioids, but high inter-individual dose-response variability makes plasma dosing impossible [72]. Fentanyl can be used in patients with mild to moderate renal and hepatic dysfunction.

6.3.3. Undesirable effects

Because of their diminished physiological reserves, elderly patients are more sensitive to the adverse effects of opioids. To ensure adequate pain management, it is therefore important to systematically look for the presence of adverse effects and, where possible, prevent and treat them [45]. The impact will be limited by applying the recommendations of good geriatric practice. However, emphasis will be placed on :

- Constipation, which is systematic and often already present before the introduction of the opioid, or which increases as soon as the opioid is introduced [39]. Its frequency is 30%. in a systematic review of the use of opiates for the treatment of chronic non-cancer pain in older adults (mean age range 60-73 years). The incidence of constipation is lower with buprenorphine than with morphine [73]. A laxative should be introduced from the start of opioid treatment, in addition to the usual dietary hygiene rules [74];

- nausea and vomiting are not systematic and generally disappear after a few days of treatment. The frequency of nausea and vomiting is lower with buprenorphine than with morphine [73]. Patients may be relieved by haloperidol or metoclopramide [63].

- Drowsiness, which is often aggravated by the co-prescription of other potentially sedative psychotropic drugs, requiring the dosage of the latter to be adjusted. If this occurs during treatment, renal function should be checked. [62] ;

- Urine retention, which is all the more likely if the patient has a prostate adenoma or a faecal impaction;

- confusion, hallucinations: if the recommendations for prescribing in old age are followed, these are not so frequent. Before attributing the problem to an opiate, another cause should be ruled out: bladder globe, ionic disorders, dehydration, and it should not be forgotten that unrelieved pain is also a cause of confusion [75];

- falls [76].

6.3.4. Monitoring

In the case of long-term treatment, renal function should be monitored regularly, either routinely or in the event of problems (e.g. the appearance of drowsiness during treatment). Respiratory depression is not to be feared if the prescription rules are followed. It will always be preceded by vigilance problems when oral, subcutaneous or transdermal opioids are used. Opioid treatment is therefore monitored by checking alertness and respiratory rate (RR). If the RR is 8 or less, the antidote, naloxone, should be used. A respiratory rate between 8 and 10 requires closer monitoring, stimulation and suspension of the opioid if it is administered continuously until it returns to 12 or more [77].

6.3.5. Opioid rotation

Switching opioids is a therapeutic strategy aimed at replacing one strong opioid with another, or changing the galenic form or route of administration, with a view to improving the benefit/risk ratio and quality of life (table III) [78, 79].

Table III: Relative analgesic equivalences of strong opioids [78, 79].

Type de rotation	Ratio relatif *
Morphine orale à hydromorphone oral	5 : 1
Morphine orale à oxycodone oral	2 : 1
Oxycodone oral à morphine orale	1: 1.5
Morphine orale à fentanyl transdermique	Se référer aux données du fabricant
Morphine sous-cutanée à fentanyl sous-cutané	70 : 1
Morphine orale à méthadone orale	5 : 1 à 10 :1 voir d'avantage selon le dosage initial

Indications that a change of opiordes is necessary:

• inadequate analgesia despite increased dosage ;

-the onset of troublesome side effects at the start of treatment or when the dose is increased dosage not controlled by symptomatic treatments [62].
A group of experts recently issued a number of recommendations designed to reduce the risks of overdose associated with rotation [80].

✓Step 1 involves calculating the daily equianalgesic dose of the new opioid.

✓Step 2 involves an automatic dose reduction of 25% to 50%, depending on the characteristics of the patient and the opioid chosen. This second step is justified by the fact that current equianalgesic doses underestimate the true potency of the new opioid, due to individual variations and the impact of incomplete cross-tolerance during chronic opioid treatment. For example, a high reduction will be applied in an elderly patient, of non Caucasian patients who are more sensitive to opioids, on high doses of an opioid at the time of rotation, or with renal insufficiency. A smaller reduction will be applied to a patient who has been on opioid treatment for a short time and/or at a low dose.

There are two exceptions to stage 2. In the case of rotation to methadone, the reduction is 75-90%. When switching to transdermal fentanyl, no reduction is necessary, as the analgesic equivalents proposed by the pharmaceutical industry include a safety factor from the outset. Step 3 involves fine-tuning the dose calculated in step 2, by assessing the intensity of pain and other medical and psychosocial factors likely to influence the likelihood of a satisfactory analgesic response and/or the occurrence of side effects. While in most cases this third step does not result in any change to the previously calculated dose, it may in some cases suggest a reduction or increase in the dosage of 15 to 30%. For example, it may be appropriate to cancel the 25% reduction in step 2 in a patient with severe pain. On the other hand, it may be justified to apply a further reduction in dosage in a pain-free, multi-medicated patient with an acute confusional state.These recommendations are intended to reduce the risk of overdose associated with opioid rotation. They provide no guarantee that the initial dose of the new opioid is appropriate. Consequently, it is essential to consider a stage 4, corresponding to daily monitoring of the patient until satisfactory pain relief is achieved, by telephone for example if the patient is at home or in a long-stay hospital. Short-acting reserve doses, equivalent to 5-15% of the daily dose, may be prescribed to compensate for inadequate dosing. The sum of the reserve doses used over 24 hours and the base treatment gives the new daily dosage.

6.4.Co-analgesics or adjuvant analgesics

Adjuvant analgesics have been defined as drugs whose primary indication is not the treatment of pain, but which possess analgesic properties under certain conditions [81]. The term "adjuvant" means that these drugs are usually used in combination with analgesics to increase their efficacy. However, the term "adjuvant" has recently been called into question because the primary indication for some of these drugs is pain management, and many are effective when used alone [82].

6.4.1. Antidepressants

a- Tricyclic antidepressants

The analgesic efficacy of tricyclic antidepressants has been established for several types of pain often encountered in elderly patients (e.g. post-herpetic neuralgia, diabetic neuropathy). Unfortunately, the use of these agents in elderly patients is limited by numerous adverse effects, including anticholinergic effects (dry mouth, constipation, blurred vision, urinary retention), cognitive changes (acute confusional state, memory disorders), cardiovascular toxicity (orthostatic hypotension, tachycardia) and an increased risk of falls and fractures [83].

Secondary amines (nortriptyline, desipramine) appear to have similar analgesic efficacy to tertiary amines (amitriptyline, imipramine, doxepin) and are better tolerated in elderly patients [84], making them a better choice if a tricyclic antidepressant is used. The elimination half-life of tricyclic antidepressants is increased 3 to 4-fold in elderly patients due to changes in hepatic metabolism (oxidation). The free fraction is also increased in the presence of hypoalbuminemia, which is common in elderly patients, and this may have clinical repercussions given their high protein binding rate (90-98%). For all these reasons, the use of tricyclic antidepressants should be avoided in elderly patients, and reserved for those who do not respond to other adjuvant analgesics with a better adverse-effect profile [54].

b- Serotonin and noradrenaline reuptake inhibitors

Venlafaxine and duloxetine have been shown to be effective for neuropathic pain. There are more data supporting the efficacy of duloxetine, which can also relieve pain and improve cognition in elderly patients suffering from major depression [85, 86], with an analgesic effect present at doses lower than antidepressant doses [86].

Venlafaxine and duloxetine are both usually well tolerated in elderly patients, without the need for dose reduction [85, 87]. They therefore represent a good alternative to tricyclic antidepressants for elderly patients with neuropathic pain and/or concomitant depression.

Elimination of duloxetine is slightly reduced with age, while venlafaxine levels are slightly higher in elderly patients [88]. When prescribing duloxetine or venlafaxine, however, attention should be paid to pharmacokinetic drug interactions involving cytochrome CYP2D6, of which duloxetine is a moderate inhibitor and venlafaxine a weak inhibitor.

c-Selective serotonin reuptake inhibitors (SSRIs)

They are usually recommended for elderly patients with depression due to their low incidence of adverse effects. Citalopram offers the advantage of a lower risk of pharmacokinetic interactions due to its minimal inhibition of CYP450. Although their elimination is reduced in elderly subjects, they are generally well tolerated [78, 79, 83]. However, their analgesic efficacy has not been clearly demonstrated.

Fluoxetine should be avoided as it is frequently associated with adverse effects due to the long half-life of the parent compound and its active metabolite (norfluoxetine) (2 and 7 days, respectively) [83]. The use of antidepressants (especially SSRIs) has repeatedly been associated with an increased risk of falls. Fall prevention strategies should always be used when an antidepressant is prescribed to an elderly patient [89].

6.4.2. Anticonvulsants

Because of their analgesic efficacy for several types of neuropathic pain, their good tolerability and the absence of pharmacokinetic drug interactions, gabapentin and pregabalin are usually recommended as first-line treatments for neuropathic pain, especially in elderly patients with multiple comorbidities and polymedication [90, 91]. Pregabalin appears to be as effective in elderly patients as in younger patients. [92] and is well tolerated [93]. The most common side effects include drowsiness, dizziness, gait disturbances and peripheral oedema. These symptoms sometimes resolve spontaneously after a few days, and can be avoided by using small starting doses and increasing the dose slowly, while closely monitoring the occurrence of undesirable effects [83].

Because of their renal elimination and the frequent decrease in renal function in elderly patients, they often respond to doses lower than the usual therapeutic doses and can rarely tolerate an increase to the maximum dose. Higher plasma concentrations of pregabalin have been observed in older subjects [94]. Although several other anticonvulsants have been shown to be effective for neuropathic pain, the frequent occurrence of adverse effects, especially with phenytoin and carbamazepine, limits their use. They should therefore be restricted to the treatment of neuropathic pain that is refractory to better-tolerated analgesics.

6.4.3. General rules of use

For systemic treatments, titration is necessary because of the wide inter-individual variability and the often poor tolerance of these drugs in old age, particularly in cognitive terms. It is usual to start with the lowest doses, regardless of the compound chosen, to increase the dose progressively in stages that vary with the time taken for the product to take effect, depending on efficacy and tolerance, and then to monitor tolerance on a regular basis once efficacy has been achieved [95]. However, depending on the compounds concerned, their onset of action may be delayed by several days to several weeks, and their efficacy on the various pain symptoms described may vary. Treatment should then be stopped gradually, to avoid abrupt withdrawal.

7.CONCLUSION

In around 70% of cases, cancer pain in the elderly may be related to the disease itself, to its treatment or to the care associated with this oncological disease, or to any other co-morbidity, which is common in this elderly population. Management of these patients is always comprehensive, combining general measures with specific drug and non-drug therapies.

In all cases, depending on the level of care desired by the patient and supported by the geriatric assessment, cancer-specific treatment remains the reference treatment for pain related to the disease itself.

This oncological treatment can be envisaged either as a cure or as a symptomatic treatment, while regularly reassessing the patient's symptomatic and functional benefits in terms of pain relief, as well as the undesirable effects of these treatments. These specific anti-cancer treatments are varied, and can be either medicinal (chemotherapy, immunotherapy or other targeted therapy), physical (radiotherapy) or surgical.If etiological treatment is not appropriate in the management of the patient, or in any case to supplement the analgesic effect of the latter, the three WHO levels of analgesics will be indicated. Their prescription, which is purely symptomatic, is based in oncogeriatrics on the same rules as for any other patient.

These analgesics will therefore be administered starting with level 1 (paracetamol), then in the event of ineffectiveness, easily moving on to level 3 analgesics (opioid treatments).

In an oncological context, and particularly when the pain being treated is related to the tumour disease, there is very little place for tier 2 analgesics, with the possible exception of buprenorphine. Buprenorphine's role in elderly patients lies in its purely hepatic metabolism, which makes it the drug of choice in cases where the pain is related to tumour disease. renal failure. The principles of prescribing Tier 3 drugs are based on titration, which means finding the minimum effective dose according to the "start low, go slow" formula. To achieve this, start with very low doses (generally ½ but up to ¼ of the recommended dose in young adults), no more than 6 times a day. Although morphine remains the drug of choice, it may be replaced by another opioid in certain cases.

This rotation may be justified by certain characteristics of the pain (oxycodone recognised in mixed nociceptive/neuropathic pain), or in cases of organ failure (fentanyl indicated in renal failure), or in order to choose a more suitable route of administration (fentanyl patch), or to obtain greater analgesic potency (hydromorphone) in rare cases in elderly patients with high minimum effective doses. Similarly, the preferred route of administration remains the oral route, which may be replaced by parenteral (iv or sc), transcutaneous or transmucosal routes when the clinical context so requires. Medication management for neuropathic pain is the same as for young patients, but with dosages adapted according to renal and hepatic function.

The reference drugs recommended as first-line treatment are still anti-epileptic drugs (gabapentin, pregabalin), followed by tricyclic antidepressants, which are not always well tolerated, particularly neuropsychologically, in elderly patients.In the context of oncogeriatrics, corticosteroids are obviously an essential part of this analgesic strategy, in the hypothesis of controlling the inflammatory component of the pain. In fact, the most recent meta-analyses do not allow us to conclude that corticosteroids have a pure analgesic effect with a good level of evidence, but the indication for corticosteroids is still recognised, particularly in the case of neuropathic pain caused by compression (of the spinal cord or peripheral nerves) or headaches caused by intracranial hypertension, as well as their overall stimulant and orexigenic effect, which indirectly influences the response to the rest of the analgesic treatment.We should also mention the specific role of anti-osteoclastic drugs such as bisphosphonates in the treatment and prevention of bone pain caused by metastases. They do not have an immediate effect, but there is evidence in the literature of real medium-term benefit, justifying their use both for analgesic purposes and to delay the onset of bone pain. The use of nitrous oxide (MEOPA), including in elderly patients, is well recognised in the context of pain during treatment or other invasive procedures. For example, this technique makes it possible to perform complex, hyperalgesic wound care in conditions of comfort that are much more acceptable to the patient, avoiding the need to use excessive doses of opiates in reserve.On a more technical note, the elderly cancer patient may also be a good candidate for surgical techniques (vertebroplasty, cementoplasty), radio-interventional techniques, or possibly loco-regional anaesthetic blocks, depending on the overall geriatric assessment and prior prognostic reflection, for specific lesions and with the aim of functional benefit.

The indications for these techniques need to be assessed on a case-by-case basis, in a collegial and above all interdisciplinary spirit.In some cases, it may be necessary to combine purely analgesic treatments with anxiolytics in order to control this symptom more completely. Despite their side-effects and potential impact on alertness, benzodiazepines remain the drug class of choice in these cases. The preferred method is to choose the compound according to its half-life (6-12 hours: Alprazolam; 10-20 hours: Lorazepam) and adapt the dose and frequency of administration to the patient's cognitive state and organ failure.Non-drug techniques are recommended in synergy with drug therapy in elderly patients.

This multimodal approach often makes it possible to avoid risky increases in drug doses in this vulnerable population. Few studies have been carried out specifically on the elderly, such as transcutaneous neurostimulation and psychotherapy (in particular cognitive behavioural therapies, the benefits of which have been shown to be greater with group rather than individual therapy). The effectiveness of hypnosis has been demonstrated in elderly subjects, but with a Mini Mental score of 25. Finally, the multiplicity of causes of this pain, and the many means available to manage it, must not interfere with a rigorous diagnostic and therapeutic approach. Thus, the need to know the precise and safe handling of analgesics or other associated molecules, which can perfectly well be offered to these vulnerable patients, is primordial, and must always be accompanied by a desire to associate multidisciplinary thinking and skills, with the aim of providing relief and preserving a level of functional skills and quality of life acceptable to the patient.

REFERENCES

1. Landi F, Onder G, Cesari M, et al. Pain management in frail, community-living elderly patients. Arch Int Med 2001; 161:2721-2724.

2. Federman AD, Litke A, Morrison RS. Association of age with analgesic use for back and joint disorders in outpatient settings. Am J Geriatr Pharmacother 2006; 4: 306-315.

3. Hwang U, Richardson LD, Sonuyi TO, Morrison RS. The effect of emergency department crowding on the management of pain in older adults with hip fracture. Amer Geriatr Soc 2006; 54: 270-275.

4. Morrison RS, Siu AL. A comparison of pain and its treatment in advanced dementia in cognitively intact patients with hip fracture. J Pain Sympt Manag 2000; 19:240-248.

5. Won A, Lapane K, Gambassi G, Bernabei R, Mor V, Lipsitz LA. Correlates and management of nonmalignant pain in the nursing home. J Amer Geriatr Soc 1999; 47: 936-942.

6. Boerlage AA, van Dijk M, Stronks DL et al. Pain prevalence and characteristics in three Dutch residential homes. Eur J Pain 2008; 12: 910-916.

7. Bosley BN, Weiner DK, Rudy TE, Granieri E. Is chronic non-malignant pain associated with decreased appetite in older adults? Preliminary evidence. J Am Geriatr Soc 2004; 52:247.

8. Rudy TE, Weiner DK, Lieber SJ, et al. The impact of chronic low back pain on older adults: a comparative study of patients and controls. Pain 2007; 131:293.

9. Blyth FM, Rochat S, Cumming RG, et al. Pain, frailty and comorbidity on

older men: the CHAMP study. Pain 2008; 140:224.

10. American Geriatrics Society Panel on Pharmacological Management of Persistent Pain in Older Persons. Pharmacological management of persistent pain in older persons. J Am Geriatr Soc 2009; 57:1331.

11. Weiner DK, Sakamoto S, Perera S, Breuer P. Chronic low back pain in older adults: prevalence, reliability, and validity of physical examination findings. J Am Geriatr Soc 2006; 54:11.

12. Culberson JW, Ziska M. Prescription drug misuse/abuse in the elderly. Geriatrics 2008; 63:22.

13. Baker KR, Nelson ME, Felson DT, et al. The efficacy of home based progressive strength training in older adults with knee osteoarthritis: a randomized controlled trial. J Rheumatol 2001;28:1655.

14. Weiner D, Karp J, Bernstein C, Morone N. Pain Medicine in Older Adults: How Should it Differ? In: Comprehensive Treatment of Chronic Pain by Medical, Interventional and Behavioral Approaches, Deer T, Ray A, Gordin V (Eds), Springer, 2012.

15. Hicks GE, Morone N, Weiner DK. Degenerative lumbar disc and facet disease in older adults: prevalence and clinical correlates. Spine 2009; 34:1301.

16. Resnick NM, Marcantonio ER. How should clinical care of the aged differ? Lancet 1997; 350:1157.

17. Weiner DK. Office management of chronic pain in the elderly. Am J Med 2007; 120:306.

18. Shi S, Mörike K, Klotz U. The clinical implications of ageing for rational drug therapy. Eur J Clin Pharmacol 2008; 64:183-199.

19. Hammerlein A, Derendorf H, Lowenthal DT. Pharmacokinetic and

pharmacodynamics changes in the elderly: Clinical implications. Clin Pharmacokin 1998; 35:49-64.

20. Tumer N, Scarpace PJ, Lowenthal DT. Geriatric pharmacology: basic and clinical considerations. Annu Rev Pharmacol Toxicol 1992; 32: 271-302.

21. Montamat SC, Cusack BJ, Vestal RE Management of drug therapy in the elderly. N Engl J Med 1989; 321:303-309.

22. Kinirons MT, Crome P. Clinical pharmacokinetics considerations in the elderly: An update, Clin Pharmacokin 1997; 33:302-312.

23. Paolisso G, Gambardella A, Balbi V, Ammendola S, D'Amore A, Varrichio M. Body composition, body fat distribution, and resting metabolic rate in healthy centenarians. Amer J Clin Nut 1995; 62:746-750.

24. Grandison MK, Boudinot FD. Age-related changes in protein binding of drugs: implications for therapy, Clin Pharmacokin 2000; 38:271-290.

25. Butler JM, Begg EJ. Free drug metabolic clearance in elderly people. Clin Pharmacokinet 2008; 47:297-321.

26. Schmucker DL. Liver function and phase I drug metabolism in the elderly: a paradox. Drugs Aging 2001; 18:837-851.

27. Mallet L. Age-related changes in renal function and clinical implications for drug therapy. J Geriatr Drug Ther 1991; 5:5-29.

28. Cockcroft DW, Gault MH. Prediction of creatinine clearance from serum creatinine. Nephron 1976; 16:31-41.

29. Nolan L, O'Malley K. Prescribing for the elderly. Part I: Sensitivity of the elderly to adverse drug reactions. J Amer Geriatr Soc 1988; 32:142-149.

30. Weiner DK, Herr K. Comprehensive Assessment and Interdisciplinary Treatment Planning: An Integrative Overview. In: Persistent Pain in Older

Adults: An Interdisciplinary Guide for Treatment, Weiner DK, Herr K, Rudy T (Eds), Springer Publishing Company, New York 2002. p.18.

31. Abdulla A, Adams N, Bone M, Elliott AM, Gaffin J, Jones D,et al. Guidance on the management of pain in older people.Age Ageing 2013;42:57.

32. Rapo-Pylkkö S, Haanpää M, Liira H. Neuropathic pain among community-dwelling older people: a clini-cal study in Finland. Drugs Aging 2015;32:737-42.

33. Chronic neuropathic pain: diagnosis, assessment and treatment in ambulatory medicine. Recommendations for clinical practice of the Société franc¸aise d'étudeet traitement de la douleur (SFETD). Doul Eval Diagn Traitement 2010;11:3-21.

34. Lutgendorf SK, Lang EV, Berbaum KS, Russell D, Ber-baum ML, Logan H, et al. Effects of age on res-ponsiveness to adjunct hypnotic analgesia during inva-sive medical procedures. Psychosom Med 2007;69:191-9.

35. Ardigo S, Herrmann FR, Moret V, Déramé L, Giannelli S, Gold G,et al. Hypnosis can reduce pain in hospitalized older patients:a randomized controlled study. BMC Geriatr 2016;16(1):14.

36. Niknejad B, Bolier R, Henderson CR Jr, et al. Association Between Psychological Interventions and Chronic Pain Outcomes in Older Adults: A Systematic Review and Meta- analysis. JAMA Intern Med 2018; 178:830.

37. Qaseem A, Wilt TJ, McLean RM, et al. Noninvasive Treatments for Acute, Subacute, and Chronic Low Back Pain: A Clinical Practice Guideline From the American College of Physicians. Ann Intern Med 2017; 166:514.

38. Morone NE, Greco CM, Moore CG, et al. A Mind-Body Program for Older Adults With Chronic Low Back Pain: A Randomized Clinical Trial. JAMA

Intern Med 2016; 176:329.

39. Jarrell JF, Vilos GA, Allaire C, Burgess S, Fortin C, Gerwin R et al. Multidisciplinary expert consensus in pain and geriatrics: use of analgesics in the management of pain in the elderly (excluding anaesthesia). J Obstet Gynaecol Can. 2018 ;40 (11):788-836.

40. Lussier D. AGS guidelines on persistent pain in older persons:lack of specific pharmacotherapeutic recommendations. J Am Geriatr Soc 2003;51(6):883-4.

41. http://www.ansm.sante.fr/.

42. da Costa BR, Reichenbach S, Keller N, Nartey L, Wandel S, JüniP, et al. Effectiveness of non-steroidal anti-inflammatory drugsfor the treatment of pain in knee and hip osteoarthritis: a net-work meta-analysis. Lancet 2016;387(10033):2093-105.

43. Machado GC, Maher CG, Ferreira PH, Pinheiro MB, Lin CW,Day RO, et al. Efficacy and safety of paracetamol for spinalpain and osteoarthritis: systematic review and meta-analysisof randomised placebo controlled trials. BMJ 2015;350:1225.

44. Roberts E, Delgado Nunes V, Buckner S, Latchem S,Constanti M, Miller P, et al. Paracetamol: not as safe as we thought? A systematic literature review of observational studies. Ann Rheum Dis 2016;75(3):552-9.

45. Pain and the elderly. UPSA Pain Institute. 2010 edition

46. Benson GD, Koff RS, Tolman KG. The therapeutic use of acetaminophen in patients with liver disease. Am J Ther2005;12(2):133-41.

47. Parra D, Beckey NP, Stevens GR. The effect of acetaminophen on the international normalized ratio in patients stabilized on warfarin therapy.

Pharmacotherapy 2007;27(5):675-83.

48. American Geriatrics Society Panel on Pharmacological Management of Persistent Pain in Older Persons. Pharmacological management of persistent pain in older persons. J Am Geriatr Soc 2009;57(8):1331-46.

49. Gloth FM 3rd. Pharmacological management of persistent pain in older persons: focus on opioids and nonopioids. J Pain 2011; 12:S14.

50. Scheiman JM, Hindley CE. Strategies to optimize treatment with NSAIDs in patients at risk for gastrointestinal and cardiovascular adverse events. Clin Ther 2010; 32:667.

51. Moore RA, Derry S, Phillips CJ, et al. Nonsteroidal anti-inflammatory drugs (NSAIDs), cyxlooxygenase-2 selective inhibitors (coxibs) and gastrointestinal harm: review of clinical trials and clinical practice. BMC Musculoskeletal Disord2006;7:79.

52. Coxib and traditional NSAID Trialists' (CNT) Collaboration, Bhala N, Emberson J, et al. Vascular and upper gastrointestinal effects of non-steroidal anti-inflammatory drugs: meta- analyses of individual participant data from randomised trials. Lancet 2013; 382:769.

53. Pickering G. Analgesic use in the older person. Curr OpinSupport Palliat Care 2012;6(2):207- 12.

54. AGS Panel on Pharmacological Management of Persistent Pain in Older Persons. Pharmacological management of persistent pain in older persons. J Am Geriatr Soc 2009; 57:1331-46.

55. Rodger K, Greasley-Adams C, Hodge Z, Reynish E. Expert opi-nion on the management of pain in hospitalized older patientswith cognitive impairment: a mixed methods analysis of anational survey. BMC Geriatr 2015;15:56.

56. Bertin P, Becquemont L, Corruble E, Derumeaux G, Falissard B,Hanon O, et al. The therapeutic management of chronic pain in ambulatory care patients aged 65 and over in France: the SAGES Cohort. Baseline data. J Nutr Health Aging 2013;17(8):681-6.

57. Clot-Faybesse P, et al. Analgesic consumption in nursing homes: observational study about 99 nursing homes. Geriatr Psychol Neuropsychiatr Vieil 2017;15(1):25-34.

58. Use of strong opioids in chronic non-cancer pain in adults - Recommendations for good clinical practice by formalised consensus. SFETD; 2016.

59. Likar R, Wittels M, Molnar M, Kager I, Ziervogel G, Sittl R. Pharmacokinetic and pharmacodynamic properties of tramadol IR and SR in elderly patients: A prospective, age-group- controlled study. Clin Ther 2006; 28: 2022-2039.

60. Beaulieu AD, Peloso PM, Haraoui B, et al. Once-daily, controlled-release tramadol and sustained- release diclofenac relieve chronic pain due to osteoarthritis: a randomized controlled trial. Pain Res Manag 2008; 13:103-110.

61. Pergolizzi J, Böger RH, Budd K, et al. Opioids and the management of chronic severe pain in the elderly: Consensus statement of an International Expert Panel with focus on the six clinically most often used World Health Organization step III opioids (buprenorphine, fentanyl, hydromorphone, methadone, morphine, oxycodone). Pain Pract 2008; 8:287-313.

62. Guerriero F. Guidance on opioids prescribing for the mana-gement of persistent non-cancer pain in older adults. WorldJ Clin Cases 2017;5(3):73-81.

63. Caraceni A, Hanks G, Kaasa S, Bennett MI, Brunelli C,Cherny N, et al. Use of opioid analgesics in the treat-ment of cancer pain: evidence-based

recommendations from the EAPC, 2012. Lancet Oncol 2012;13(2):e58-68.

64. Moisset X, Trouvin AP, Tran VT, et al. Use of strong opioids in chronic non-cancer pain in adults. French recommendations for good clinical practice by formalised consensus (SFETD). Presse Med 2016;45:447-62.

65. Naples GJ, Gellad WF, Hanion JT. Managing painin older adults: the role of Opioid Analgesics.ClinGeratrMed 016;32(4):725-35.

66. King S, Forbes K, Hanks GW, et al. A systematic review of the use of opioid medication for those with moderate to severe cancer pain and renal impairment: a European Palliative Care Research Collaborative opioid guidelines project. Palliat Med 2011; 25:525.

67. Arnstein P. Balancing analgesic efficacy with safety concerns in the older patient. Pain Manag Nurs 2010; 11:S11.

68. Heiskanen T, Mätzke S, Haakana S, et al. Transdermal fentanyl in cachectic cancer patients. Pain 2009; 144:218.

69. Vadivelu N, Hines RL. Management of chronic pain in the elderly: focus on transdermal buprenorphine. Clin Interv Aging 2008; 3:421.

70. Payne R. Opioid pharmacotherapy. In: Berger AM, Portenoy RK, Weissman DE, editors. Principles and Practice of Palliative Care and Supportive Oncology, 2nd edition, Philadelphia: Lippincott Williams & Wilkins, 2002, 68-83.

71. Dosa DM, Dore DD, Mor V, Teno JM. Frequency of long-acting opioid analgesic initiation in opioid-naive nursing home residents. J Pain Symptom Manage 2009; 38:515.

72. Gupta DK, Avram MJ. Rational opioid dosing in the elderly: dose and dosing interval when initiating opioid therapy. Clin Pharmacol Ther 2012; 91:339.

73. Walsh SL, Preston KL, Stitzer ML, et al. Clinical pharmacology of buprenorphine: ceiling effects at high doses. Clin Pharmacol Ther 1994; 55:569.

74. Papaleontiou M, Henderson CR Jr, Turner BJ, et al. Outcomes associated with opioid use in the treatment of chronic noncancer pain in older adults: a systematic review and meta-analysis. J Am Geriatr Soc 2010; 58:1353.

75. Vella-Brincat J, Macleod AD. Adverse effects of opioids on the central nervous systems of palliative care patients. J Pain Palliat Care Pharmacother 2007; 21:15.

76. Weiner DK, Hanlon JT, Studenski SA. Effects of central nervous system polypharmacy on falls liability in community-dwelling elderly. Gerontology 1998; 44:217.

77. Zutler M, Holty JE. Opioids, sleep, and sleep-disordered breathing. Curr Pharm Des 2011; 17:1443.

78. Mercadante S, Caraceni A. Conversion ratios for opioid switching in the treatment of cancer pain: a systematic review. Palliat Med 2011; 25: 504-515

79. Knotkova H, Fine PG, Portenoy RK. Opioid rotation: The science and the limitations of the equianalgesic dose table. J Pain Symptom Manage 2009; 38: 426-439

80. Fine PG, Portenoy RK: For the ad hoc expert panel on evidence review and guidelines for opioid rotation. Establishing "Best practices" for opioid rotation: Conclusions of an expert panel. J Pain Symptom Manage 2009; 38: 418-424

81. Lussier D, Portenoy RK. Adjuvant analgesics in pain management. In: Doyle D, Hanks G, Cherny N, et al, eds. Oxford Textbook of Palliative Medicine, Third Edition. Oxford, England: Oxford University Press, 2003; 349-377.

82. Lussier D, Beaulieu P. Toward a rational taxonomy of analgesic drugs. In: Beaulieu P, Lussier D, Porreca F, Dickenson AH, eds. Pharmacology of Pain. Seattle: IASP Press, 2010, 27- 40.

83. Lotrich FE, Pollock BG. Aging and clinical pharmacology: implications for antidepressants. J Clin Pharmacol 2005; 45: 1106-1122.

84. Pickering G, Marcoux M, Chapiro S, David L, Rat P,Michel M, et al. An algorithm for neuropathic pain mana-gement in older people. Drugs Aging 2016;33:575-83.

85. Raskin J, Wiltse CG, Siegal A, et al. Efficacy of duloxetine on cognition, depression, and pain in elderly patients with major depressive disorder: an 8-week, double-blind, placebo- controlled trial. Am J Psychiatr 2007;164:900-909.

86. Raskin J, Xu JY, Kadasz DK. Time to response for duloxetine 60 mg once daily versus placebo in elderly patients with major depressive disorder. Intern Psychogeriatr 2007; 20:309-327.

87. Wasan AD, Ossanna MJ, Raskin J, et al. Safety and efficacy of duloxetine in the treatment of diabetic peripheral neuropathic pain in older patients. Curr Drug Saf 2009; 4:22-29.

88. Skinner MH, Kuan HY, Skerjanec A, et al. Effect of age on the pharmacokinetics of duloxetine in women. Br J Clin Pharmacol 2004; 57:54-61.

89. Kerse N, Flicker L, Pfaff JJ, et al. Falls, depression and antidepressants in later life: a large primary care appraisal. PLoS ONE 2008; 3:e2423.

90. Gore M, Sadosky A, Leslie D, Sheehan AH. Selecting an appropriate medication for treating neuropathic pain in patients with diabetes: a study using the U.K. and Germany Mediplus Databases. Pain Pract 2008; 8:253-262.

91. Wehling M. Multimorbidity and polypharmacy: how to reduce the harmful

drug load and yet add needed drugs in the elderly? Proposal of a new drug classification: fit for the aged. J Am Geriatr Soc 2009; 57:560-561.

92. Sharma U, McCarberg W, Young JH, LaMoreaux L. Pregabalin treatment for neuropathic pain: efficacy and tolerability in older people. J Pain 2005; 3(Suppl. 1):S29.

93. Montgomery S, Chatamra K, Pauer L, Whalen E, Baldinetti F. Efficacy and safety of pregabalin in elderly people with generalised anxiety disorder. Br J Psychiat 2008; 193:389-394.

94. May TW, Rambeck B, Neb R, Jürgens U. Serum concentrations of pregabalin in patients with epilepsy: the influence of dose, age, and comedication. Ther Drug Monit 2007; 29:789-794.

95. Hanon O, Jeandel C. Guide PAPA. Medication prescriptions adapted to the elderly. PharmHosp Clin 2015;51(4):376-7.

SUMMARY

In around 70% of cases, cancer pain in the elderly can be linked either to the disease itself, or to the treatments or care associated with this oncological disease, or to any other co-morbidity, which is common in this elderly population.

The management of these patients is always comprehensive, combining general measures with specific drug and non-drug therapies. In all cases, cancer-specific treatment remains the reference treatment for pain related to the disease itself.

If etiological treatment is not appropriate in the management of the patient, or in any case to supplement the analgesic effect of the latter, the three WHO levels of analgesics will be indicated. Their prescription, which is purely symptomatic, is based on the same rules in onco-geriatrics as for any other patient.

Finally, the multiplicity of causes of this pain, and the many means available to manage it, must not interfere with a rigorous diagnostic and therapeutic approach. Thus, the need to know the precise and safe handling of analgesics or other associated molecules, which can perfectly well be offered to these vulnerable patients, is essential, and must always be accompanied by a desire to associate multidisciplinary thinking and skills, with the aim of providing relief and preserving an acceptable level of functional skills and quality of life for the patient.

TABLE OF CONTENTS

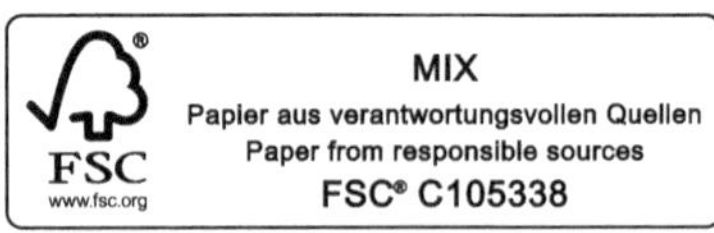

Printed by Books on Demand GmbH, Norderstedt / Germany